Better a crust of bread with love than a whole loaf without.

For all the grandmothers who have created memories of clattering dishes, bubbling pots, and meals that will remain forever in our senses.

For my niece, Vivian Magnolia, who may be the only person who loves food more than I do, and for my Nonnie who, after all these years, has me convinced that being "a great eater" is the highest compliment one can receive.

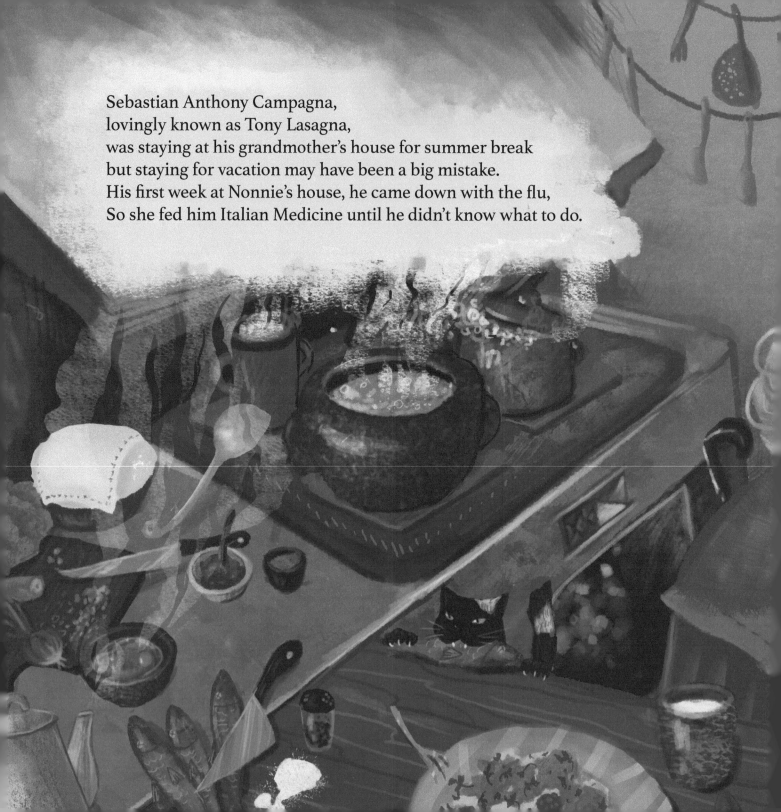

Sebastian Anthony Campagna,
lovingly known as Tony Lasagna,
was staying at his grandmother's house for summer break
but staying for vacation may have been a big mistake.
His first week at Nonnie's house, he came down with the flu,
So she fed him Italian Medicine until he didn't know what to do.

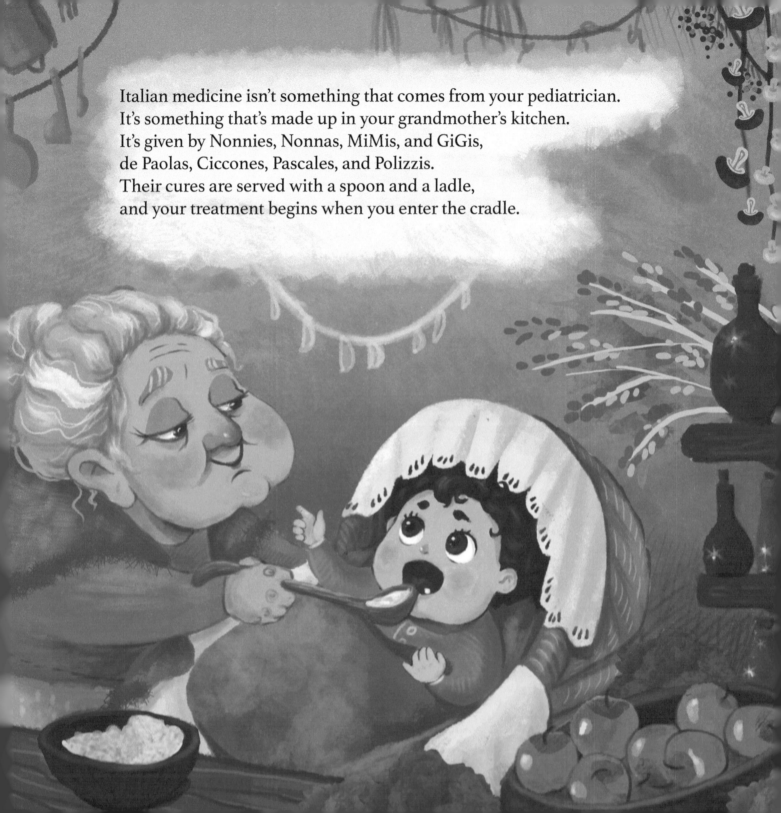

Italian medicine isn't something that comes from your pediatrician.
It's something that's made up in your grandmother's kitchen.
It's given by Nonnies, Nonnas, MiMis, and GiGis,
de Paolas, Ciccones, Pascales, and Polizzis.
Their cures are served with a spoon and a ladle,
and your treatment begins when you enter the cradle.

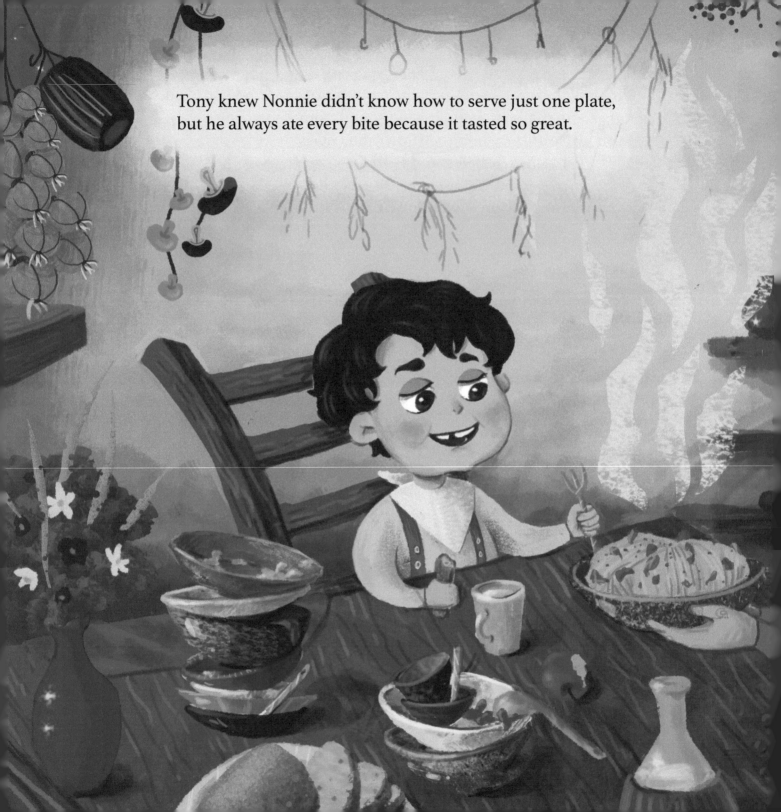

Tony knew Nonnie didn't know how to serve just one plate,
but he always ate every bite because it tasted so great.

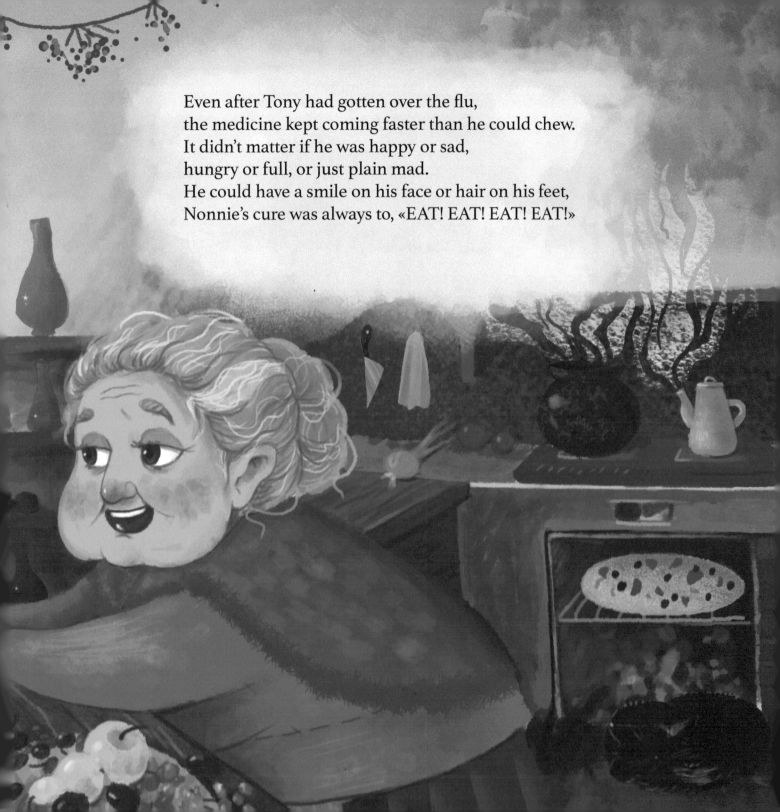

Even after Tony had gotten over the flu,
the medicine kept coming faster than he could chew.
It didn't matter if he was happy or sad,
hungry or full, or just plain mad.
He could have a smile on his face or hair on his feet,
Nonnie's cure was always to, «EAT! EAT! EAT! EAT!»

If Nonnie thought Tony was getting a case of the blues,
she'd feed him sausages until his toes swelled out of his shoes.

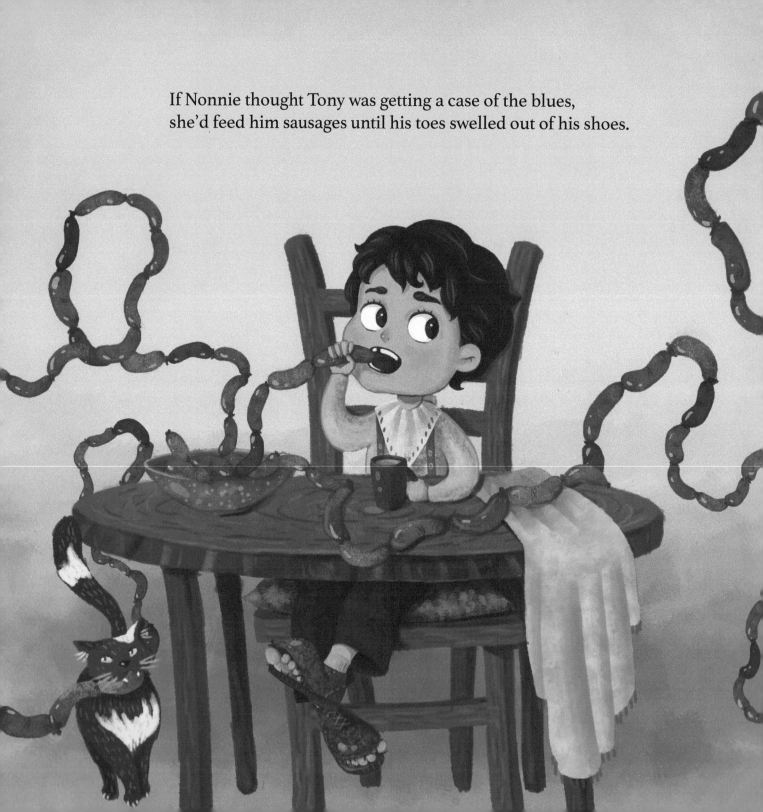

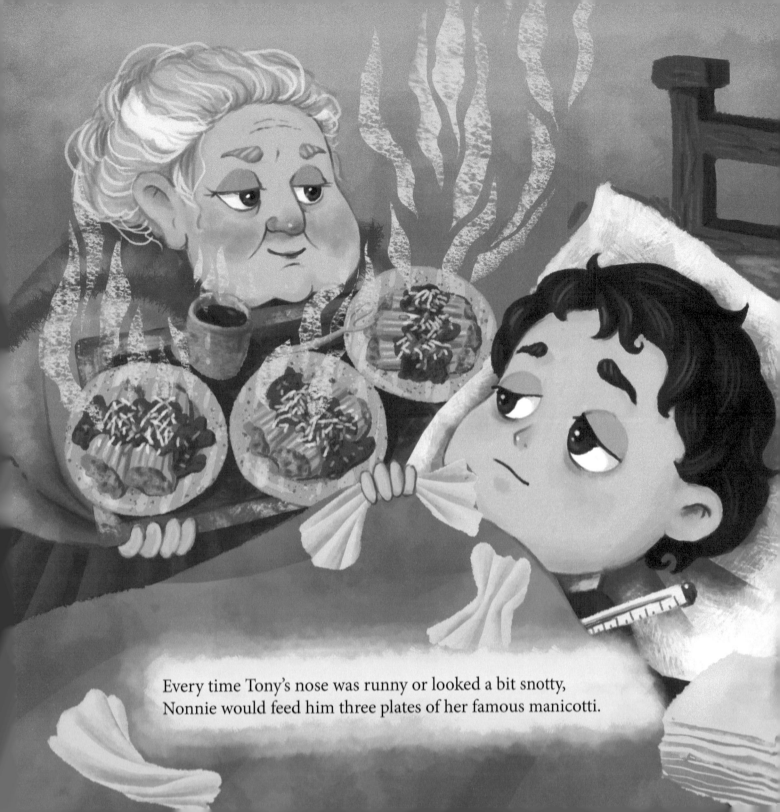

Every time Tony's nose was runny or looked a bit snotty,
Nonnie would feed him three plates of her famous manicotti.

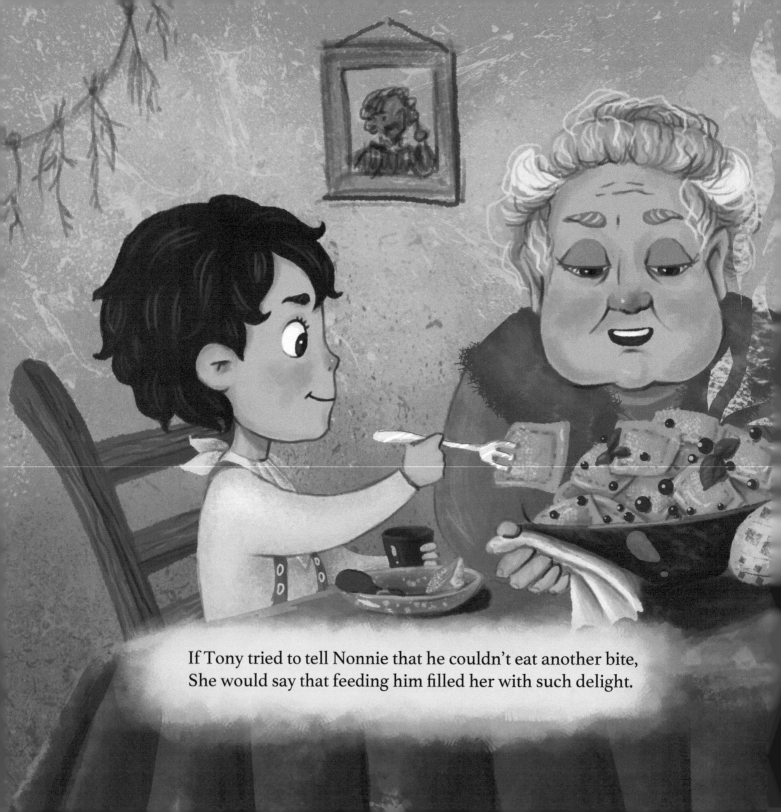

If Tony tried to tell Nonnie that he couldn't eat another bite,
She would say that feeding him filled her with such delight.

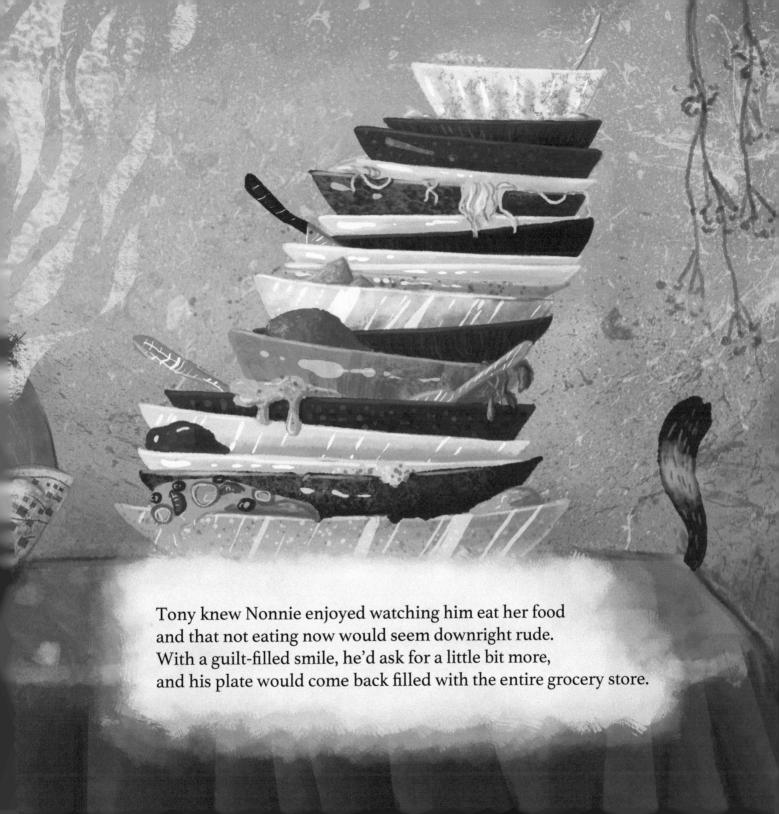

Tony knew Nonnie enjoyed watching him eat her food
and that not eating now would seem downright rude.
With a guilt-filled smile, he'd ask for a little bit more,
and his plate would come back filled with the entire grocery store.

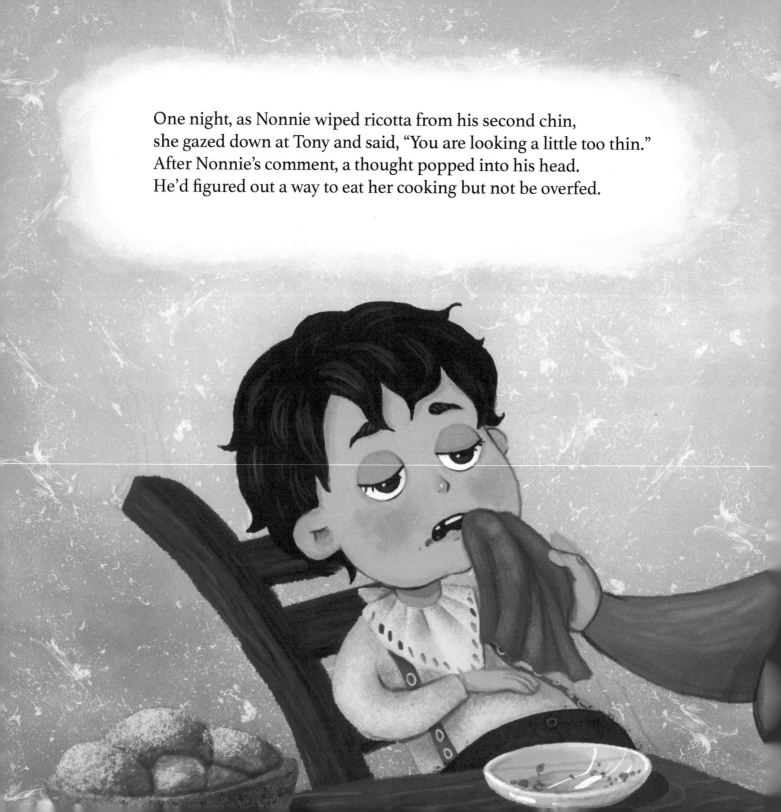

One night, as Nonnie wiped ricotta from his second chin,
she gazed down at Tony and said, "You are looking a little too thin."
After Nonnie's comment, a thought popped into his head.
He'd figured out a way to eat her cooking but not be overfed.

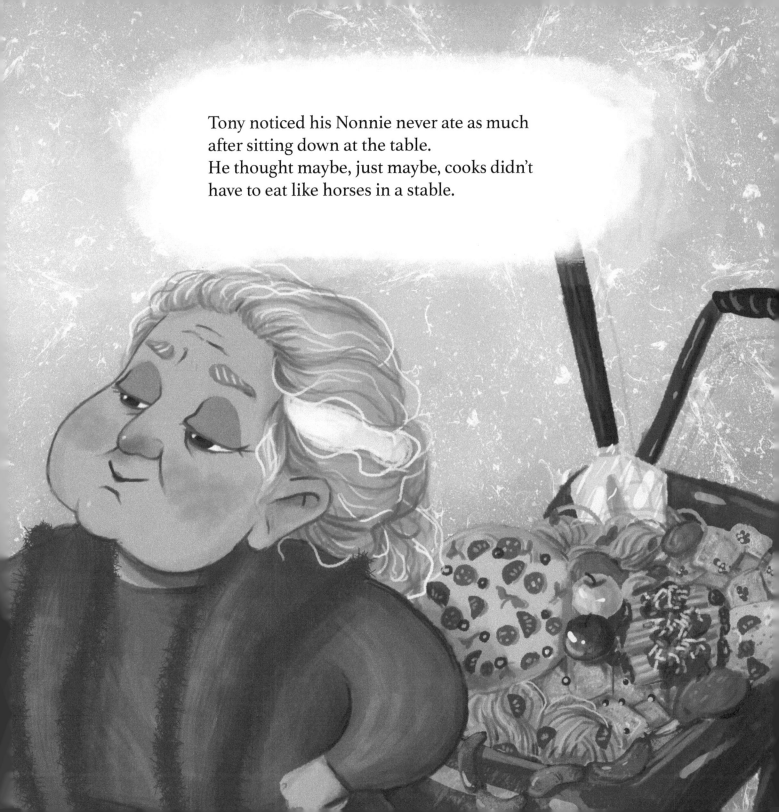

Tony noticed his Nonnie never ate as much
after sitting down at the table.
He thought maybe, just maybe, cooks didn't
have to eat like horses in a stable.

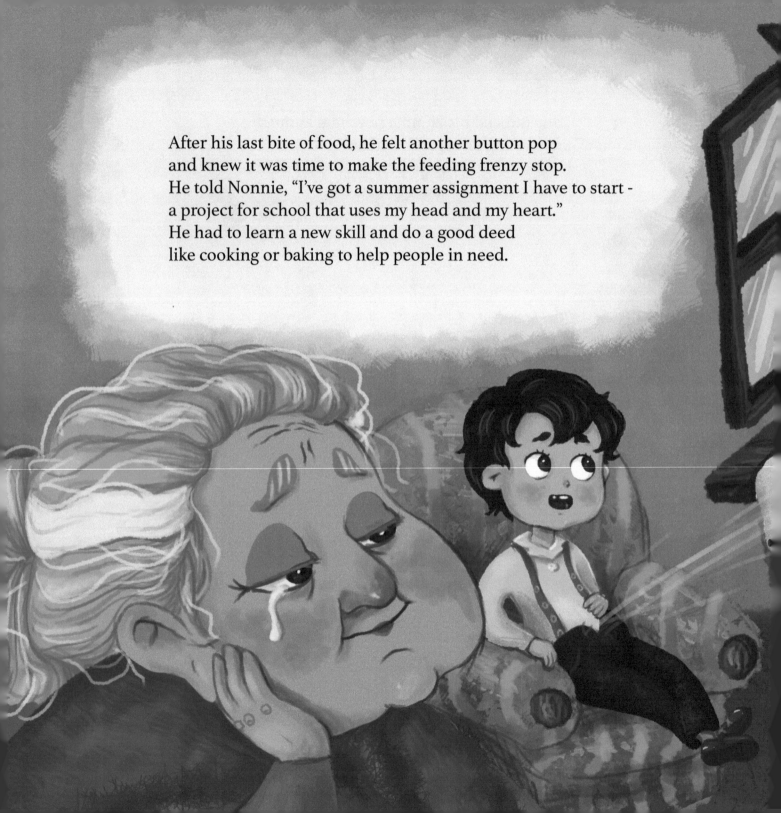

After his last bite of food, he felt another button pop
and knew it was time to make the feeding frenzy stop.
He told Nonnie, "I've got a summer assignment I have to start -
a project for school that uses my head and my heart."
He had to learn a new skill and do a good deed
like cooking or baking to help people in need.

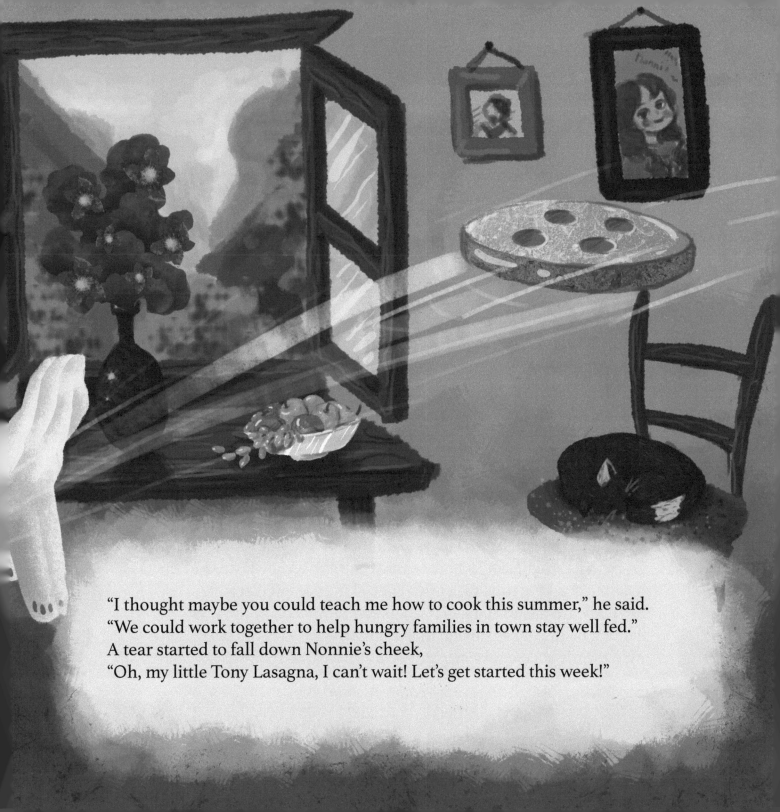

"I thought maybe you could teach me how to cook this summer," he said.
"We could work together to help hungry families in town stay well fed."
A tear started to fall down Nonnie's cheek,
"Oh, my little Tony Lasagna, I can't wait! Let's get started this week!"

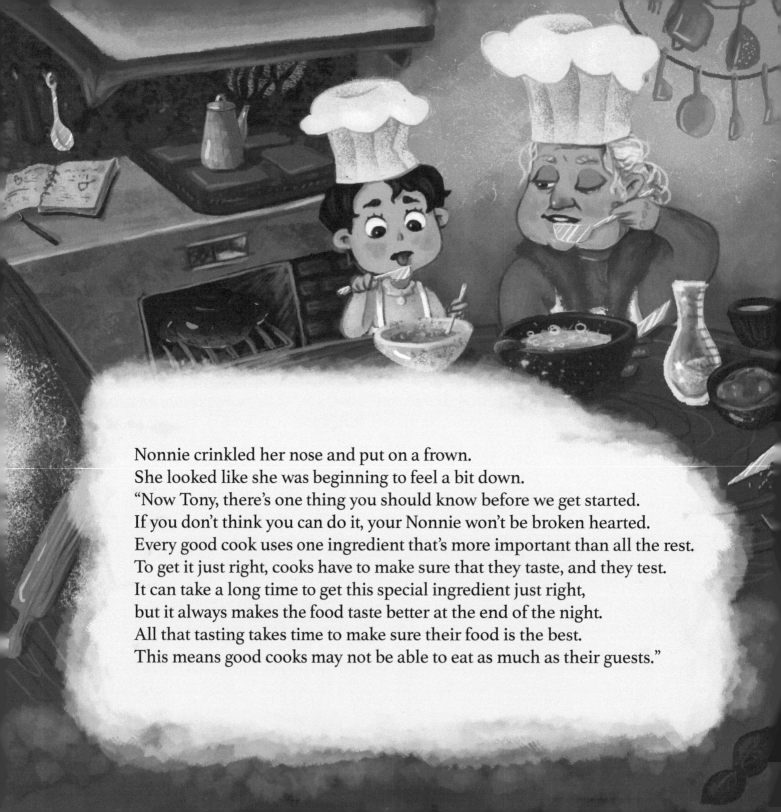

Nonnie crinkled her nose and put on a frown.
She looked like she was beginning to feel a bit down.
"Now Tony, there's one thing you should know before we get started.
If you don't think you can do it, your Nonnie won't be broken hearted.
Every good cook uses one ingredient that's more important than all the rest.
To get it just right, cooks have to make sure that they taste, and they test.
It can take a long time to get this special ingredient just right,
but it always makes the food taste better at the end of the night.
All that tasting takes time to make sure their food is the best.
This means good cooks may not be able to eat as much as their guests."

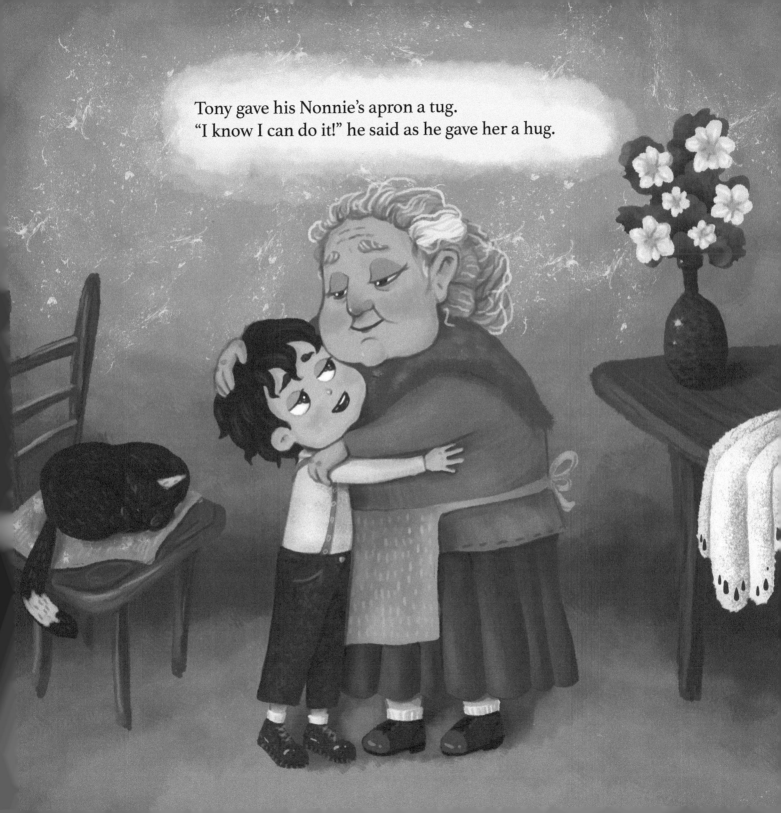

Tony gave his Nonnie's apron a tug.
"I know I can do it!" he said as he gave her a hug.

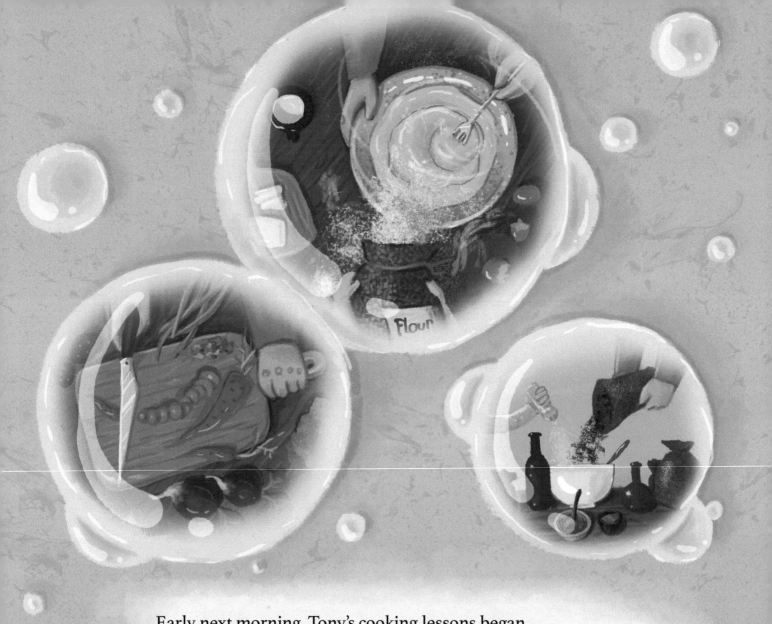

Early next morning, Tony's cooking lessons began.
He was amazed at all that could be done with just a pot and a pan.
They seasoned, they stirred, they measured, they mashed.
They mixed, they sifted, they pinched, and they dashed.

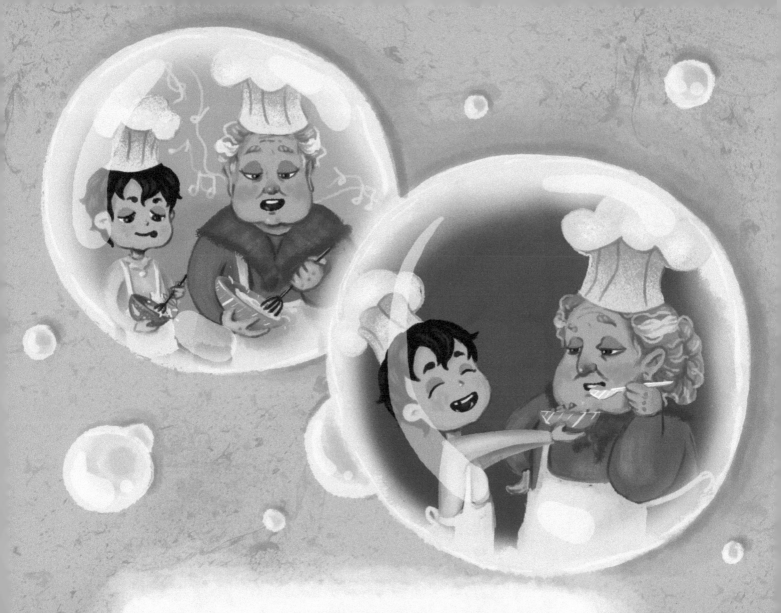

They tasted, they tested, they baked, and they boiled.
They smiled, they laughed, and they sang while they toiled.
By the time that their Sunday family dinner drew near,
Tony was ready to cook with his Nonnie without any fear.

They made Cousin Teddy five plates of spaghetti,
because lately he had been feeling a little unsteady.

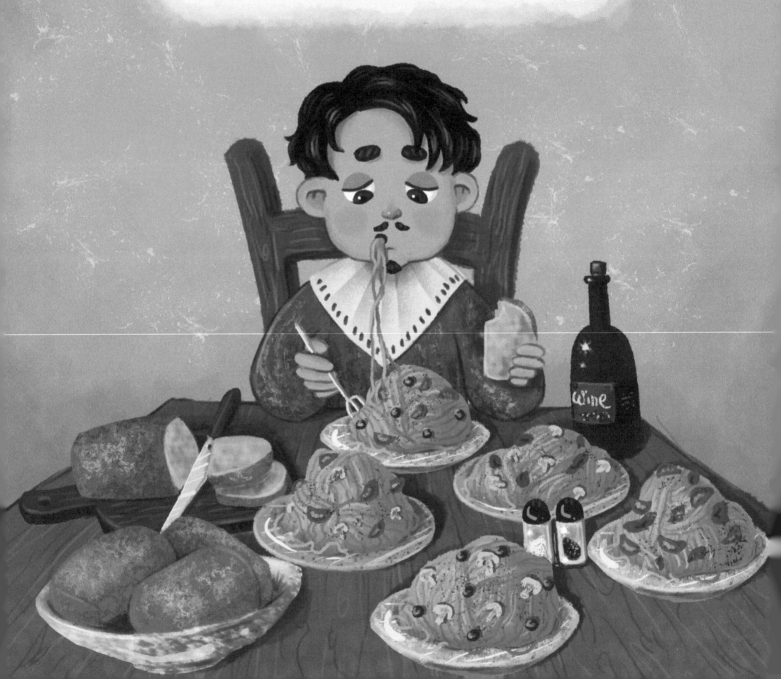

When Aunt DeeDee said, "My eyes are tired and beady."
The cooks whipped up two platters of Nonnie's meaty baked ziti.
When Cousin Betty's waistline looked just a bit too teeny,
Out came a wheelbarrow full of creamy fettuccini.

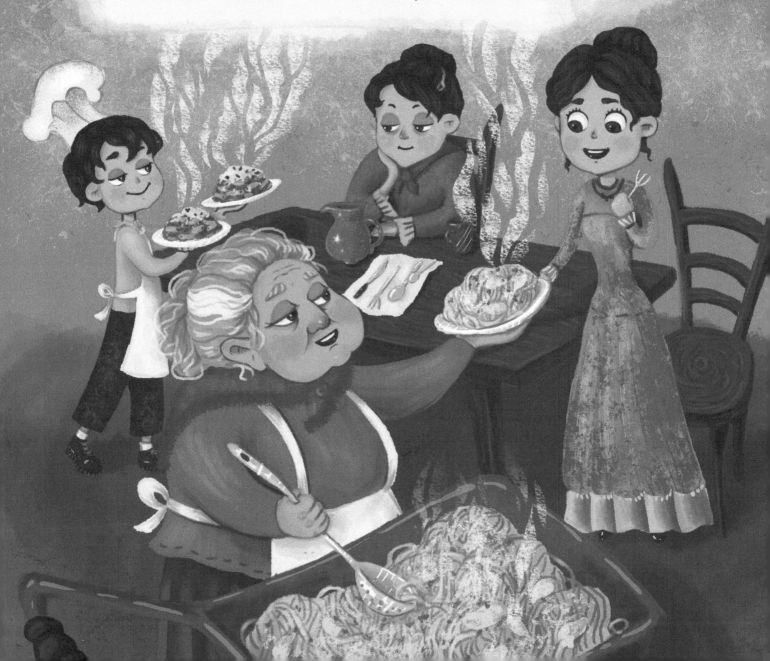

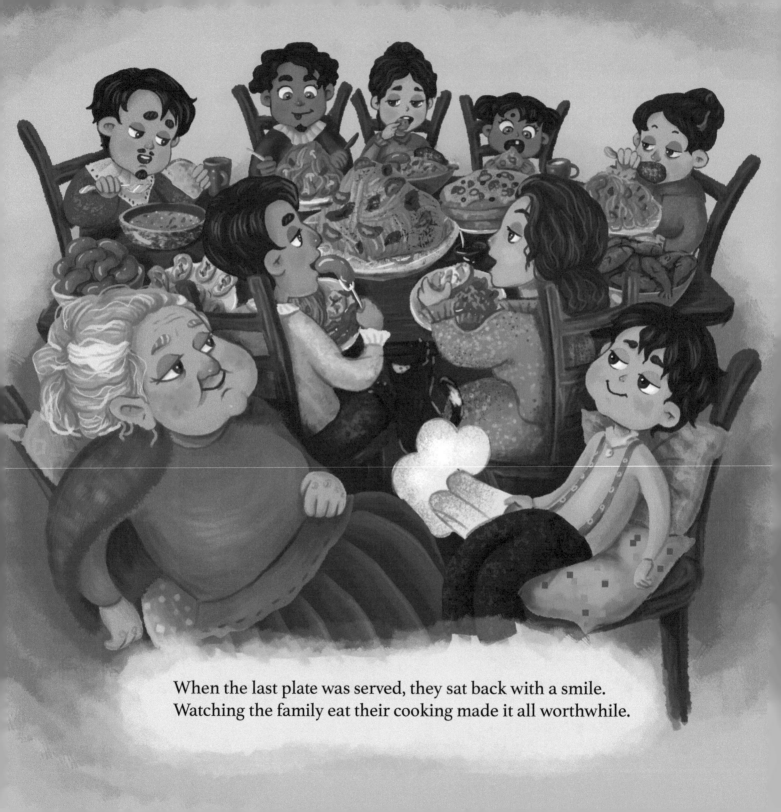

When the last plate was served, they sat back with a smile.
Watching the family eat their cooking made it all worthwhile.

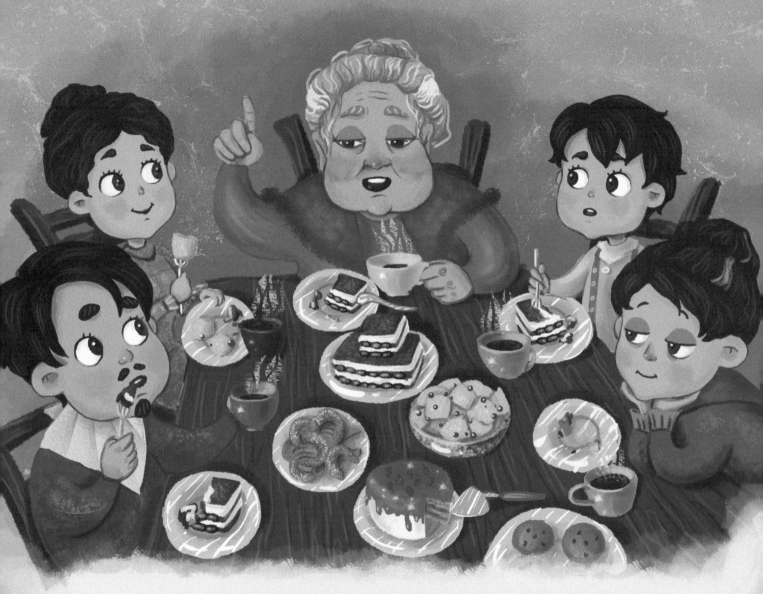

Nonnie told the family about the school project and about Tony's new plan –
How they wanted to cook meals down at the shelter, once a week if they can.
Everyone listened to Nonnie while they sipped coffee and ate tiramisu.
After she'd finished, the entire family declared, "We want to help too!"

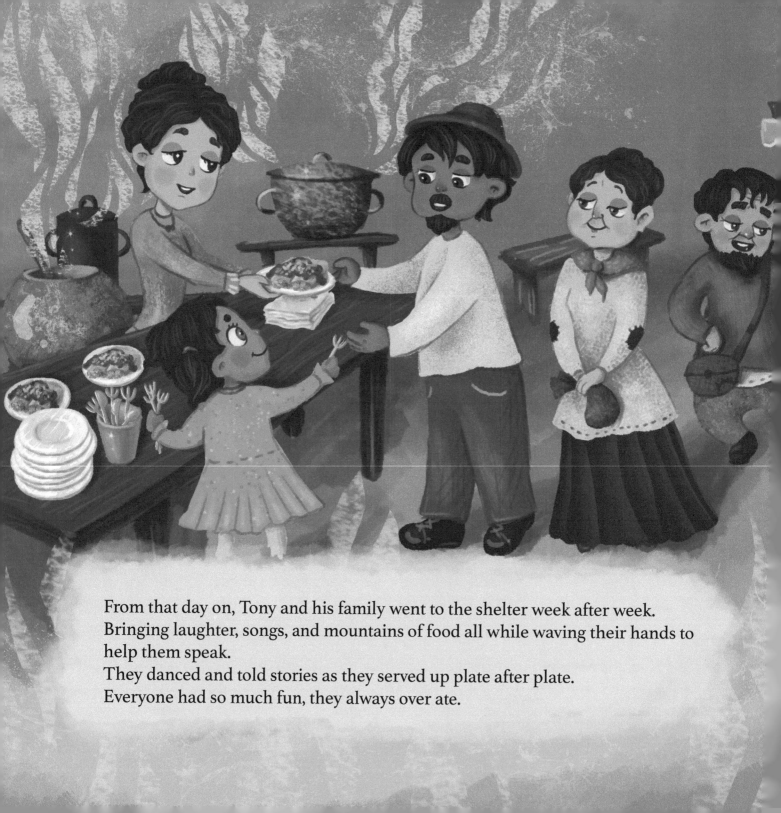

From that day on, Tony and his family went to the shelter week after week.
Bringing laughter, songs, and mountains of food all while waving their hands to
help them speak.
They danced and told stories as they served up plate after plate.
Everyone had so much fun, they always over ate.

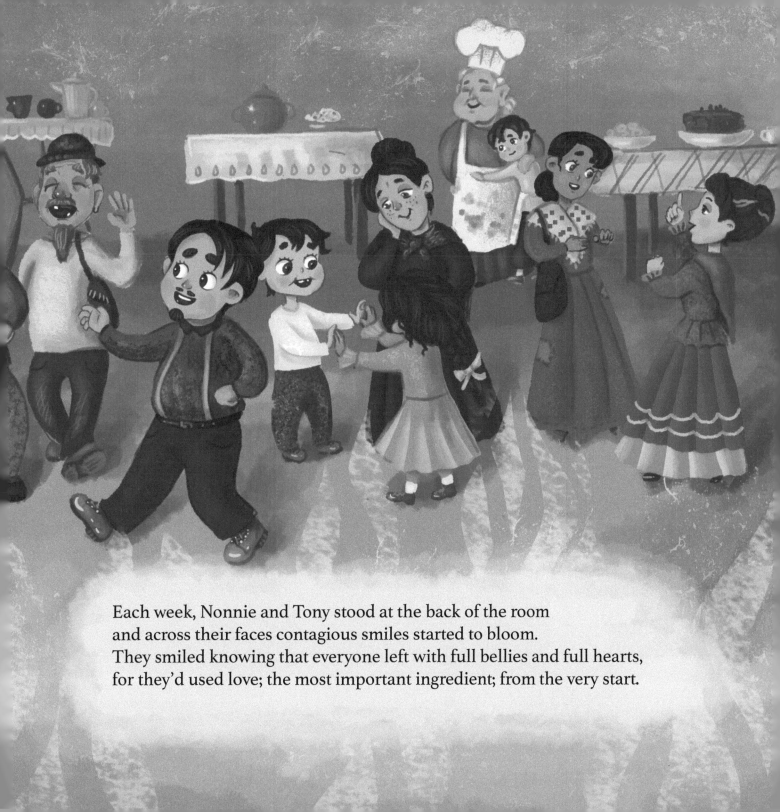

Each week, Nonnie and Tony stood at the back of the room
and across their faces contagious smiles started to bloom.
They smiled knowing that everyone left with full bellies and full hearts,
for they'd used love; the most important ingredient; from the very start.

A Portion of the profits from this book go to DC Central Kitchen.

ABOUT DC CENTRAL KITCHEN

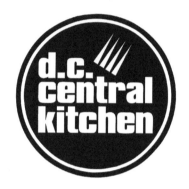

DC Central Kitchen (DCCK) is an iconic nonprofit and social enterprise that combats hunger and poverty through job training and job creation. Our approach provides hands-on culinary job training while creating living-wage jobs and bringing nutritious, dignified food where it is most needed in our city. We serve scratch-cooked farm-to-school meals in DC schools; deliver fresh, affordable produce to corner stores in neighborhoods without supermarkets; provide delicious catering; and operate fast-casual cafes. DCCK has been featured in national media including The Washington Post, The Atlantic, National Geographic, PBS NewsHour, and more. To learn more, visit dccentralkitchen. org or follow @dccentralkitchen on Instagram.

About the Author

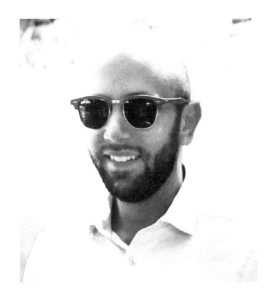

When Zach was growing up, his mother always took her four kids to the library and made reading a huge part of their lives. His favorite days were when she would have them climb out of their bedroom window onto the roof and read them books under the branches of their Black Walnut tree. These memories have stuck with him and are the reason he is an avid reader and writer today. Zach hopes to impart that same passion upon a new generation of children through his stories.

Zach graduated from Radford University in 2006. He currently lives with his lovely wife, Johanna, in Manassas, Virginia. He is the author of Fleeting Moments, a poetry book co-authored with his father, and four children's books: Italian Medicine, The Story of the Snugglefink, The Return of Foggitytree, and The City of Paws2Care. When not reading or writing Zach can be found hiking in the woods, where he is regularly mistaken for a sasquatch.

www.zacharytamer.com

About the Illustrator

Yevheniia Melnyk is an illustrator from Kiev, Ukraine. Her great-grandmother taught her how to cook when she was a child, just like Tony. As a child, she mastered the secrets of cooking national, and family dishes. Her great-grandmother had a superpower - everything she cooked turned out to be incredibly tasty. Along with the recipes, she received a lot of wise advice from her great-grandmother. Yevheniia recalls this time with warmth in her heart.

CPSIA information can be obtained
at www.ICGtesting.com
Printed in the USA
BVHW021648120521
607125BV00002B/10

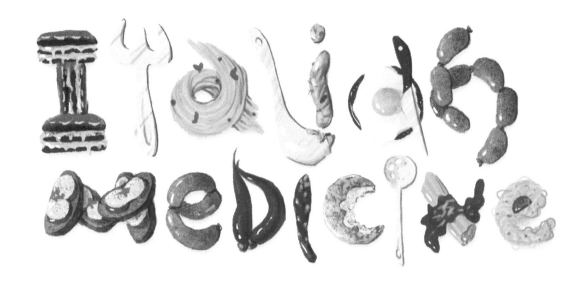

Italian Medicine

By Zachary Tamer

Illustrated by Yevheniia Melnyk

ISBN: 978-1-7368268-0-5